Praise for A LIFE INTERRUPTED

"Reader: You will be TRANSFORMED BY INJURY—vicariously and literally as you read this book of poems.

"There is a message in this poetry that is poignant and essential for all who are recovering from traumatic brain injury and for those who love them. This poetry will transform you: Mind, Body and Spirit. You will feel your skin prickle; your heart and lungs open and your mind relax in a way that prose would never penetrate. You will become aware of the greater importance of your Life experience, transformed by injury. You will know the stages and transitions that occur on the healing journey with Traumatic Brain Injury. You will experience a wakeup call mentally and spiritually to declare the purpose of your life. As you read *A Life Interrupted,* you will be interrupted to become more authentic and whole, while wholly different than before.

"This book should be required for every neurologist graduating from residency. It should be in every VA hospital for soldiers returning from War. It should be at the bedside of all who suffer at home. A caretaker should gently read these words out loud to heal and be healed.

"The book not only outlines the TBI journey but specifies resources for healing. The best of the best therapy and therapists in this country are listed at the end of the book. These approaches hold hope for all who have chosen this challenging and difficult life in transition. To those who work with TBI and those such as Louise Mathewson who live beyond it, we owe our gratitude and awe."

LINDA W. PETERSON-ST. PIERRE, PH.D.
Emeritus Professor, University of Nevada School of Medicine
Marriage & Family Therapist
Author of *Children in Distress: A Guide for Screening Children's Art,*
Clear Vision: The Power of Story & *Write Out Loud: A Guide for*
Families who Live and Work in War and War-Like Environments

"A car accident left Louise Mathewson with a traumatic brain injury (TBI) that changed her forever. She awoke after a two-week coma unable to walk, read, speak, remember. But something deep inside had not been touched—her essence, her soul, remained intact. It struggled through the confusion and chaos to reclaim its voice as she struggled to regain her physical and mental abilities. This book of short poems recounts Louise's strenuous journey back from the darkness of this 'invisible injury' and allows us to rejoice with her when, finally, she is able to change her personal understanding of TBI to 'transformed by brain injury.'"

BARBARA STAHURA, C.J.F.
author of
After Brain Injury: Telling Your Story
www.barbarastahura.com

"A must-read for anyone in the traumatic brain injury (TBI) field. This poetry is packed with inspiring words painting a patient's viewpoint of the long journey from horrific accident to revitalized person. Louise is constantly viewing her injury as the glass half full, finding new possibilities in day to day happenings while re-developing brain pathways. In her words, 'TBI = transformed by injury.'"

DEBORAH ZELINSKY, O.D.
www.mindeyeconnection.com

"In few words, in poetic metaphor, readers are thrown into the realities of brain injury and recovery in ways that will stay with us for a long time. Louise Mathewson's writing is a map to a journey we may not all take, but we all need to understand! I am grateful for the comprehendible guidance of Louise's writing—it increases my understanding and allows me to be a better companion to people with traumatic brain injury however and wherever our paths cross."

CHRISTINA BALDWIN, M.S.,
author of
*Storycatcher: Making Sense of Our Lives through
the Power and Practice of Story*

"After a severe traumatic brain injury a life is changed; the recovery will be challenging, but the soul need not be lost. Louise Mathewson has created an amazing collection of insights into brain injury recovery as a transformation, one that can be experienced in terms of a positive journey. In her words, she has truly 'Learned to dance with an injured brain.'"

JULIE STAPLETON, M.D.
Neurotrauma Specialist
Boulder, CO

"A Life Interrupted by Louise Mathewson is a collection of uplifting poetry written in the first person but easily transferable to the reader. The metaphors and multiple modalities of rich imagery gently move the reader forward from one page to the next. The intimacy she is able to share with the reader and deeply optimistic sense of faith is inspiring for any and all who have experienced loss....Her personal story is one that should be shared with anyone with a brain injury."

ROBERT G. KOHN, D.O.
Diplomate Neurology American Board of Psychiatry & Neurology
Assistant Clinical Professor Radiology
University of Illinois-Chicago
www.DrRobertKohn.com

"The poetry here is piercing, all the more so when you realize it opens a window to a landscape rarely charted. Certainly not charted with such power by a poet whose brain, as she writes, once was 'sheared.' Louise Mathewson was lost, was hijacked, when her brain hit a dashboard in a horrific car accident. She made her way out of the 'dungeon of despair' one word, one stanza, at a time. And so we all emerge from *A Life Interrupted,* forever wiser, forever more grateful for the grace of the everyday."

BARBARA MAHANY
reporter & feature writer
www.barbaramahany.com

"Brain injured individuals are launched into a journey through unfamiliar and chaotic terrain, a path with few signposts and one mostly traveled alone. Many enter that wilderness and do not return. Louise Mathewson has traveled that path. Yet, remarkably, she has refused to surrender to its isolation. Through her poetry she insists that we join her there as she wrestles with the angel of transformation, as she emerges from the cocoon of her grief to become the shimmering poetic butterfly so evidently here now. What emerges through her writing is an evocation of the experience of brain injury that is by turns wrenching, detailed, clinically accurate, ruthlessly honest, and in the end spiritually rich and nourishing.

"This is not necessarily an easy book to read. Much of it is about the peculiar qualities of suffering and distress that happen to people following a traumatic brain injury. This is not the breezy, Hollywood version of life we are so accustomed to, where bad things never happen to good people. Here is the voice of a good person, and something quite bad has clearly happened. Louise refuses to let herself or us off the hook too easily. 'You must look at this,' she seems to be saying; 'this is real and it's not okay to ignore it.' So we must accompany her on the journey of her personal tragedy and ultimate transformation.

"A wonderful jewel of a book!"

DARELL M. SHAFFER, M.D.
Hearthstone Institute
www.hearthstoneinstitute.com

A LIFE INTERRUPTED

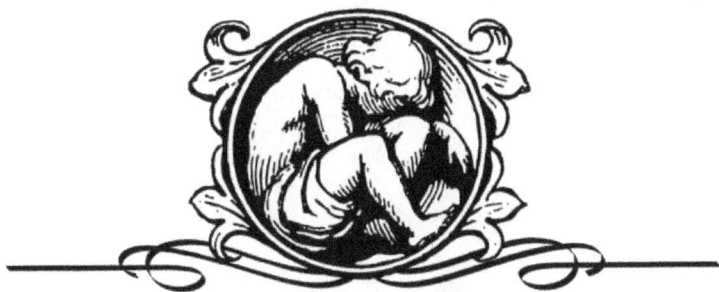

Living With Brain Injury

Louise Mathewson

PEARLSONG PRESS
NASHVILLE, TN

Pearlsong Press
P.O. Box 58065
Nashville, TN 37205
www.pearlsong.com
www.pearlsongpress.com

Cover illustration by Carol Mathewson.
Book & cover design by Zelda Pudding.

Trade paperback ISBN: 9781597190558
Ebook ISBN: 9781597190565

"Life After Brain Injury" won Honorable Mention in the 2008
Inglis House Poetry Contest. "A Road Not Chosen" was originally
published in *Breath and Shadow Magazine,* Fall/Winter 2008. "Lost"
and "A New Day" were originally published in *Wordgathering: Journal
of Disability Poetry,* September 2007.

Library of Congress Cataloging-in-Publication Data

Mathewson, Louise, 1947–
 A life interrupted : living with brain injury / Louise Mathewson.
    p. cm.
 ISBN 978-1-59719-055-8 (original trade pbk. : alk. paper)—ISBN
978-1-59719-056-5 (ebook)
 1. Mathewson, Louise, 1947—Poetry. 2. Brain—Wounds and
injuries—Patients—Rehabilitation—Poetry. I. Title.
 PS3613.A8434L54 2012
 811'.6—dc23

                              2012012269

Acknowledgements

A LIFE INTERRUPTED: LIVING WITH BRAIN INJURY is the story of my long journey through the experience of traumatic brain injury following an auto accident. At the moment of impact, my world was forever changed. Rebuilding my life and discovering a new Self has been a spiritual walkabout—taking me through a myriad of emotions and seemingly insurmountable challenges, but ultimately bringing me to a place of renewed hope, gratitude and grace.

I wish to thank the following individuals, who have each contributed to my recovery and allowed me to tell my story through the publication of this book:

My husband, Stu, for his undying support, love and loyalty through a near-death state, recovery therapies, difficult grief, and then through the changes in me. My children, Terri and Mike, and their spouses, Rob and Lisa, for traveling from New York City and Minnesota to Boulder to stand by me in those early days, for their love, concern, and care for me as I healed, and for their acceptance of the changes in me as their mother. My sister, Terre, for her honesty, love, care and support of my husband at a time when he couldn't think clearly to ask questions. My brothers, John and Chuck, for their love and concern through my recovery. My sisters- and brothers-in-law, friends, and California in-laws for their support, in particular their prayers of love and healing. My sister-in-law, Carol Mathewson, with appreciation for her creation of the beautiful cover illustration for this book.

Boulder Community Hospital (BCH) for the excellent nursing care I received while in ICU. Pam Nettro, research nurse of the neuro-trauma unit, for overseeing my care and for educating nurses and my family about brain injury care. David Kenney, chaplain at BCH, for his support of my husband through this very difficult time. Dr. Julie Stapleton, Mary Dineen, and the rest of the rehab therapy team who oversaw my therapies and cared for me.

My publisher, Peggy Elam of Pearlsong Press, for believing in the message of my work. Rachel Moritz, for her compassionate help in preparing for publication. Gayle Nosal, poetry therapist, for her writing workshops and support before the accident, and for her coaching in the months following. Linda Leedy Schneider for her amazing support, mentoring, coaching, encouragement, and sage advice as I grow as a poet. Barbara Delage for her wise and heart-filled guidance in the publishing and marketing process.

...and to the angel who spoke to me while I was in a coma and gave me reassurance that there was a purpose for this trauma.

Thank you, God,
for sending an angel with a message
that traumas are about transformation.

LOUISE MATHEWSON

CONTENTS

AFTER THE CAR WRECK

My spirit,
shook up
in a car of chaos,
lost
in a sea of space,
forgot
who I am,
where I was,
how I lived,
expressed life.

Floundering,
I fell down a tunnel
into
a valley of dread
where infantile demons
racked my soul
through a dark night.

Pieces

My life in pieces

scat
ter
ed

among shards of glass
twisted metal
piece
s

of
the puzzle
of my life
thrown
u
p
in the air
lying on the ground of life
wait
ing
to be put back together.

Climbed Another Mountain

I climbed
another mountain,
emerged from an accident.

Car totaled,
my forehead slashed,
eyelid cut,
brain shirred,
bruised,
as it bounced back and forth
inside my bony skull.

Cells, neurons
stretched out of shape
no longer work as they once did.
Thoughts must
find new neurons
to relay their messages
to my body.

A Computer Crash

Our computer's
hard drive
crashed one day.
It accepted
no data,
processed
no information,
gave out
no details,
had no working memory.

Like the day
our car crashed
and my head
hit the dashboard,
my brain injured, sending
me into outer space,
the hard driver that I was
forced to rest,
receive
from spirit and my angels.

No thoughts,
no processing necessary,
just breathing,
receiving air,
rest,

relax,
have a break,
take it easy,
unwind from
my control tower.

I had to
let go and let God
do the rest.

Life Was Interrupted

I hear an announcement
in the dark of a sleep-coma

assurance
from
above,
as an angel speaks:

"This is about transformation."

Time out,
take a rest.

A chance to sift through old scars,
remove the scabs of old beliefs
that mar my future.

I wait
as each scab is removed
by a wave of tears
that washes another level of soul.

I must protect,
like a baby's skin,
each new layer
of fresh, soft
soul-skin.

I Remember Little

of ICU.
I do remember
my daughter Terri's eyes,
goblets of love,
my son Mike's hand,
the soft touch of God.

I remember a little
of my hospital room—
looking out at a red brick wall.
All bricks looked the same
as the days of my life did then.

I remember women
sitting at my side—
some read,
some knitted.
None talked much to me.
I was in and out of sleep.
I didn't know enough to ask why they were there.
They didn't seem to be doctors or nurses.
I learned later they were there
to watch me, make sure I didn't get up.

I remember
sips of water.
Nurses held the cup for me to drink.

I couldn't get enough.
I remember
being fed applesauce.
I wasn't hungry till I tasted
the sauce.
Then I wanted more
but was allowed only a few spoonfuls.

I remember
being taken in a wheelchair
to a lab.
They took pictures
of my brain
to see—
if the bleeding inside my skull had stopped.

I Didn't Know

I didn't know
I couldn't move my left side

I didn't know
I couldn't walk

I didn't know
I couldn't breathe on my own

I didn't know
I couldn't eat

I didn't know
I couldn't swallow

I didn't know
I couldn't remember the day before

Then they took me
off the ventilator
unhooked the catheter
gave me sips of water
fed me applesauce with a spoon

Later
I rode in an ambulance
to the rehab hospital

I didn't understand
that it was my second ride in an ambulance

There at the rehab hospital—

I didn't know
I couldn't walk without a walker

I didn't know
I had no sense of balance
I walked into walls

I didn't know
I wasn't supposed to get out of bed alone
when I did
an alarm sounded

I didn't know
I made no sense when I talked
wondered why people left
when I wasn't finished talking

I didn't know
I couldn't hold a pen well
but I could write chicken scratch
unreadable as it was
I was embarrassed

I did remember
I used to have beautiful handwriting

LOST

I lost the map
inside my brain,
neurons stretched
beyond their reach.

Now, messages
stopped in their tracks
can't find their way.
They must discover
other routes
to make connections.

New roads
need to be created.
A fresh map
must be drawn.

A New Day

It's a brand new day,
just woke
from a coma,
been gone
so long,
knocked out-
side myself,
how to get back:
the task
before me.

I am
pure
consciousness,
spirit
separated
from her vessel.
I yearn to come back
all the way
to my toes,
set them upon
this hallowed ground.

Every day
I get to try
to come back.
My purpose now

to come home,
to knit
the pieces of my soul
together.

My skin
can't feel,
those feet, ah
they run clumsily
without me inside of them.
Legs?
What do my feet attach to?
Where is the ground?

After a Coma

Part of me
taken
taken away
not far
hovered
just above my body
lifeless.

Lost in space
another world
split
split off
less than whole
divided
from myself.

A hole in my spirit

is left

I ache

for that slice
separated
from myself.
I call her back
she doesn't want to come

I tell her
we will be better together.

She comes
the pain lessens

I begin to flower.

HIJACKED

My head
had a collision with the dashboard
forehead and eye split in pieces
blood spilled
a river down my face
it trickled warm on a cold day

knocked out
into a cocoon of coma
a hand reached in
and took apart physical memories
how to walk
write
shed tears

dismantled
mental memories
how to use the computer
process incoming information
understand some words

stole
old memories
of childhood
took bits of each
and left them with missing pieces

stole
younger memories of life as a mother
a mid-life woman with a passion for writing

stole
my sense of self
gained through years of living

hijacked
from myself
returned with a dusting off
to a clutter of chaos
to name
sort
organize
while I wipe up tears

as I recreate
a new me.

I Didn't Used to be Like This

I didn't used to forget what I just said.

I didn't used to find my memories shot full of holes.

I didn't used to get confused when people used pronouns,
have no idea what they were referring to,
what they might mean,
what we were just talking about.

I didn't used to find my brain frozen,
unable to think,
useless to process abstract concepts.

I didn't used to feel adrenalin rushes of fear
at the sound of a word, harmless as it may be.

I didn't used to feel a flood of chemicals
causing my mind to lose its way,
stop dead in its tracks, unable to move forward.

I didn't used to feel drained, unable to think,
barely able to speak after trying to understand
abstract thoughts for 10 minutes.

I didn't used to be like this;
my brain worked.

A New Chapter in Life

I lost my place
in the chapter of a book I was reading
I couldn't find my way back
I had to pick up
somewhere over the rainbow of pages
and read on.

After an injury to my brain
I lost my place
in a chapter of my life.
Hard as I tried
I couldn't find my way back
to the last line
I had written
before I was knocked out.

I searched
in books
in the darkness
under covers
out in nature.
I had to turn
to a new page
and start again,
learn new lessons
in the game of life.

A New Dance

After a car wreck
spirit crushed
psyche gashed
trauma effects took over
my body, mind and spirit.

The landscape of my life now dark.
Shaky nerves cover my skin with geyser bursts of terror
erupting along the grid of my body.

As I rest, walk, reflect, write,
stretch my circle of comfort,
I learn to dance with trauma in my cells.
I learn to dance with an injured brain.
I learn to dance new steps with life.

A Monsoon

Clouds mushroom in my head,
dark, dreary,
silent,
threatening
a storm.

I greet the cloud's power.
Then
the outer banks burst,
a hard-driving, torrential rain
floods my evening.

Confusion, muddy thoughts,
wails,
red-hot thunder claps
crash out of the silence.

A lightning bolt
of awareness
connects heaven
to earth,
lights the darkness
of a grief monsoon.

STRANGE JET LAG

My eyes
tired
energy lags
body lags
spirit lags
disoriented in time
is it 11 a.m.
or 8 p.m.
not sure
I feel
between worlds
confused
my head whirls.

Like brain injury
coma
I lost days
of my life
lagged behind myself
disoriented in life
unsure where to go
addled
hypersensitive to energy
can't depend on myself
for the first time in my life
helpless, shame, despair,
a chasm
between me and my fellow humans.

SHAME

Hemmed in
surrounded
slathered
with shaving soap
shame on my skin
clings
lathers up with the slightest touch
until I shave it off
in layers
I may cut it
as I take it off
and it will hurt
but I will have new skin that goes deep
fresh, pink with love
as I was created

A LODE OF GRIEF

My voice changes,
begins to crack,
reveals a smaller me
hidden below the surface
of the water of my life.

My voice
strikes a lode of grief,
tears
fall in streams
down the hills
of my cheeks.

Tear streams drop off
the cliff of my chin
into the stew of
my life
with a blemished brain.

The Difference Is

when I make decisions
it seems I float,
carried on a waft of air,
not by choice, you see.
My feet can't find ground
to rest upon.

The difference is
she got lost
in a car crash,
spirit
trying to find her way home.

The difference is
I trusted her,
relied on her
for everything.
Now
she is changed,
altered
to fit me in a new way,
a way I was not prepared for.

The difference is
it's a new map
with new routes I must get used to,
new friends
I must make with my brain.

I Had to Get It Out

I had to get away
from that dirty shame
reminders every day
I had to get away.

I sit here by the fountains
outside Caribou
the sound of water
soothes my psyche's wounds.

I don't know why he stays
I don't know why I wail
it aches so deep
I sob from my gut
all that pain
from so long ago
pain from now
that he'll never know
the struggle
I go through
every day
to make my brain work
to remember thoughts, ideas
I long to express.

It all comes back
to how I have hurt him

not acknowledged
his idea
I know how to sob
without making a sound
I am embarrassed to make any noise.

I come to the waters
with my paper and pen
a mocha and a book
to soothe my sorrow
to lay down my pain
in the pond.

DUNGEON OF DESPAIR

I fell in a pit
deep
way down
to the center of another world
a world I did not fit in
a world that belongs to demons.

Frightened
I grieved
asked
"How did I get here?
Will I find my way home?
Is there a way home?"

One step
another
slowly
one after the other
it's a long way up
the Sacred Mountain
from the dungeon of despair.

A DAY TO REMEMBER

It's Thursday
an anniversary, of sorts
my body remembers
my mind does not
heaviness builds in my chest
eyes fill
another wave of grief threatens
a storm
upon the ocean of my life
waves build slowly
life changed in an instant.

This story
I was told
hit from behind
our car spun on black ice
struck a guard rail
slid across the pavement
smashed into an oncoming car
my door
the target.

My head hit hard
brain bounced inside my skull
blood vessels sheared
lobes bruised
neurons stretched

beyond capacity,
safety in the world destroyed.
The old me
put to rest.

LIFE AFTER BRAIN INJURY

No one knows
how hard I struggle to find words,
to convey thoughts
in my mind—not just words, but thoughts, ideas.

No one knows
the mood swings that happen all day long inside my brain—
tears that come out of the blue,
a desire to pull back from life, yet connect with life,
but little spirit to hold that paradox
and follow the positive side.

No one knows
how it feels to be troubled over little things in life.

No one knows
how hard it is to live with catastrophic thoughts
that invade my brain all day through the day
for no reason.

No one knows
how hard it is to know my hard drive crashed
and try to reconstruct it with pieces missing.

No one knows
how it feels to have the old software of memories removed,
precious memories gone, stolen in the night.

No one knows
how it feels to have thoughts about death when my life is
blessed and I know it, but the thoughts persist.

No one knows
how it feels to have been taken away from my body,
to come back, but not be all the way in and
not be able to force myself in.

No one knows
how it feels to not remember what was just said,
to have memory that selects of its own accord
with no regard to my wishes.

No one knows
how it feels to listen to someone speak while trying to
make sense of the words and find
a hole in my brain where the processor is down,
maybe forever.

No one knows
how it is to have fatigue and know it's my brain that's tired,
nothing in the vessel of my body operates well
without my brain's assistance.

No one knows
what it is to have one's sense of God suddenly skewed
and not understand or know how to repair the warp.

No one knows
how it feels to have to recreate myself, my life at fifty-nine,
with less brain power.

When I'm all done with this new creation,
I hope I like the new me.

I will!
Because it contains my essence.

SHIVERS

run up my arms
I hunger
for a soft cocoon
lined in velvet
while cells
rearrange themselves
in my vessel
till
the angel of transformation
recreates
me—
a new
blue
butterfly
of beauty

LOSSES

Meaning
I lost it
in a car wreck
lost
but not forever.

Trust
lost
spattered like blood
drops
upon the pavement of life.

Executive skills
organization, initiation and motivation
lost
as my head hit the dashboard
control I never really had,
shattered.

Now
pieces of the puzzle of my life
wait to be put back
together
into a whole that makes sense
to a brain that can't
make judgments, decisions.

Grief
I found it
my tether to soul
will lead me back
to myself.

SCAFFOLDING

I walk
past a building
surrounded by scaffolding
covered with thick plastic.
Inside men work
to restore
an old building
renew it.

It is the same for me
after brain injury.
I surround myself
with a scaffolding of comforts
while spirit
restores itself
renews me.

An Anger Cat

"Good,"
she said,
"you let your anger cat
out of the bag!"

"I did!"
I told him,
"This is what makes me
so f…in' angry
about brain injury!
I have NO memory
of this f...in' new
insurance card!"

He walked just behind me
as I approached the pharmacist
and gave him the new card.
The pharmacist then explained
about insurance complications,
and how he'd work it out.

I didn't understand,
then turned to my husband
and said, "This is another thing
that makes me so f…in' mad
about my injury!"
I can't always process instructions.

I feel like a fool and I'm angry,
like a cat caught in a corner,
when I have to ask and ask again.

SHADOW LIFE

In the shadow
lies
infantile dragon demons
red mad monsters
crabby creatures,
sisters with wicked steps
that hide dreams
from days done
a life lived.

While
grapes grown
from seeds
in the dark,
mature
into a delicate wine
to sip and savor
in the days ahead
of a life.

MAYBE

Maybe
I don't have to
accumulate information like I have for a lifetime.

Maybe
I don't have to
process every bit of language I hear.

Maybe
I don't have to
understand it all.

Maybe
I don't have to
be the homemaker I've been for so long.

Maybe
I don't have to
be the perfect daughter, mother, wife.

Maybe
I don't have to
be what others expect me to be.

Maybe
I've been
granted freedom from the 'have-tos'

put on me by parents, society, myself.

Maybe
I can be who I am,
a person who feels energy everywhere,
sends blessings, peace and love to everyone.

Maybe
I don't have to
know the meaning of life.

Maybe
it is in living again.

AFTER

brain injury
coma
forces her to spin
dead story threads
woven
with bits of hardwood beliefs
soil particles from her previous life
cemented together with chemicals
in her brain.

She lies low
quiet
still
waits.

Sheds layers
of her worm-like
wrap.

Spirit
grows
emerges
a beautiful butterfly.

Brain Injury

granted me
coma
deep sleep
to hear my angel's voice.

Time to rest
repair shattered circuits
form a new me.

Darkness
to create
new life
as a poet.

An Account with Interest

I was carried to a place of peace and darkness,

coma.

I was put into an account
for transformation,
withdrawn from life
by an injured brain.
While in this savings account
I accrued interest.
After a couple years
heaven's teller opened the window
and words began to flow out.

My interest in life
became the power of the word.

POSSESSION

The ocean is a sea
of moods
calm, peaceful
one day,
gray, stormy
another.

Big waves slap
one another,
pound the shore
the next day.

My brain
lives in a sea of moods
after an injury.
Can't make decisions,
can't commit,
can't initiate acts
because I am possessed
by a sea of moods.

WHAT WAS LOST

I didn't know
what I lost
in the chaos
of a car accident.

Four years later
I know an earthquake
shifted the landscape of my brain
took me into the dark
to find
what was buried
of my old self.
Who I thought I was
is lost.

Dare I now be who I really am
in a world
of chaotic, and yet, creative energy?

I am a player on the stage of life.
I am a prophet.
I am a poet.

Now
I know who I am.

TRAUMA

Reined in my spirit
confidence
s
  h
     a
  t
      t
  e

     r
  e
     d

heart
brok e
n open

balance
  w
    r
      eck
  ed

trust   devour ed

faith
in
vaded

safety
stolen
in the night

my spirit
harnessed
by the demons of trauma

I find my way out
through the written word of spirit

A Road Not Chosen

A spider web
reaches
curves
arches
from one point
to different ends

f o r m s

shapes—hearts, angles, triangles
roads to the outside.

I weave a life
from stories spun
of roads taken
in my life.
One not chosen
traumatic brain injury.
When I hit my head—
hard
in a car accident
knocked out
in a coma
no one knew
what would be left of me.

I spin inwards after TBI

till I hit the center mark
golden goodness of my source.

When I get back out—
side
through the gift of poetry
I will find my way back
to the web
of life on earth.

ECLIPSED

A lunar eclipse last night
magic in the dark
the moon
covered by earth's shadow.
I too was eclipsed
by depression.

A shadow was cast
on my brain
by trauma
from an injury to my brain
in a car accident.

My spirit
pressed flat
so it can't stand up
the sadness of despair
like mud in my gas tank.

WORD ROUNDUP

the puzzle is called.
Unrelated letters float in a square,
wait to be connected
to make a word.

As I come back
to a brain rattled
by a blow to my head
I found my word recall is broken,
aphasia it's called.

Thoughts float in my head
but the page where words appear is blank.
I play word roundup
with an empty page,
no words arrive
and anxiety grows
inside my head
as I plead for my brain to work.

Who will speak for me
when my page is blank?

Comin' Back

I'm comin' back
after a car wreck
trauma to my brain
bounced around
inside its skull
I left my body.

I'm comin' back
after being gone two weeks
in a coma
where I lost memories
parts of myself.

I'm comin' back
even though
geyser bursts of terror
shoot up
at unexpected times
inside my skin.

I'm comin' back
with new dreams
after old dreams were shattered.

I'm comin' back to life.

I Reclaim My Mind from Aphasia

I reclaim
the alphabet soup
of letters that slid
down the chute into my head.

I reclaim
the Scrabble board
where I arranged letters into words.

I reclaim
wood blocks with words
that I sorted into sentences.

I reclaim
Word Roundup
puzzles
where I rounded up words
that I recognized.

I reclaim
the game of Scattergories
in which I put words that belong in a category
and organized my thoughts.

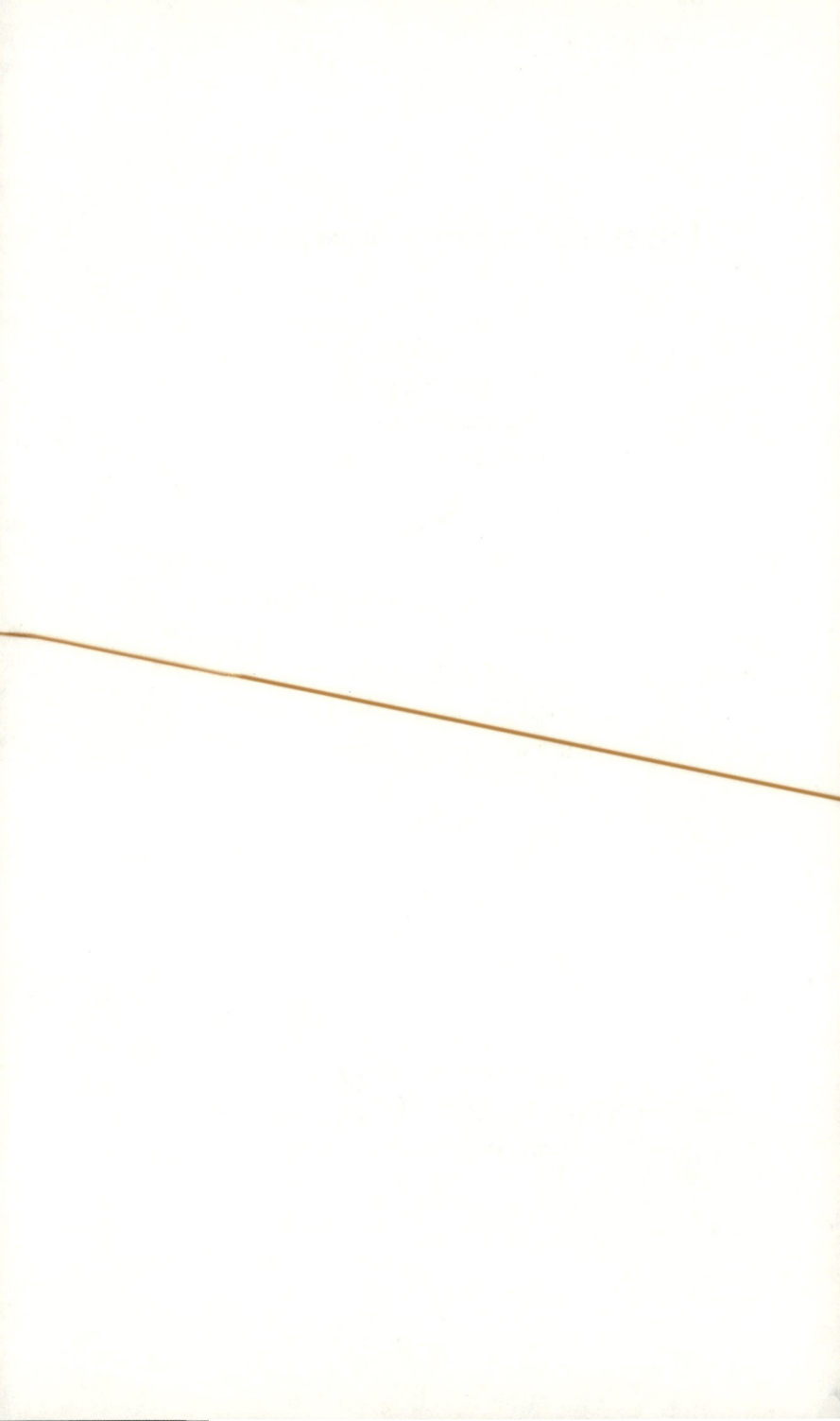

If Not

If not
for traumatic brain injury
I would not know the geography of fears
that constrict my heart.

If not
for traumatic brain injury
I would not know the darkness inside me
and the stars that twinkle, even in the dark.

If not
for traumatic brain injury
I would not know the lushness of the landscape
of my soul.

If not
for traumatic brain injury
I would not write this poem
learn ways to heal.

If not
for traumatic brain injury
I would not see my own goodness.

A WALTZ AND TANGO WITH LIFE

On a winter morning
I sit by the window
watch snowflakes whirl
and twirl
as they waltz
with the air
toward earth.
Perky and playful
as they twist and turn
this way and that.

Dancers
carried on air currents unseen
like my life
after meeting with death.

I, too, am carried on wings,
Divine wishes
for me,
this way, no that way
if I'm off-course,
even a bit.

A tango with trust at every turn.
Trust, in the lead,
wants to face fear in a duel
to shoot it in the head
so when it lands on earth
fear is dead.

A Salad of Words

She explains her mistake.
Distracted by the tilt of her head,
a gentle smile
and wave of her hand
brushing her mistake away,
I wait for my decaf.
I hear a salad of words
tumble into the bowl of space
over the counter between us,
cluttered with a tip jar, bars, candies for sale,
distractions to my damaged brain
that struggles to focus on letters
hanging unseen in the air,
and a memory that loses
every few words.

"I…mistake…check…charged…credited…
…then charged…sorry…only two cents…you get…"

I've lost myself in the salad of words,
hanging in the air.
I leave the store,
tears clouding my eyes.

I Am She Who

I am she who hugs trees,
smoothes the velvet of rose petals.

I am she who savors the scent of lilacs,
    roses and ocean breezes,
dances with the sun and warm air.

I am she who paints landscapes of life
    with the lusciousness of words,
hears her name whispered in the breezes.

I am she who listens to silence
watches eagles, hawks, heron and egrets,
wades the waves of life's wisdom.

I am she who climbs mountains of grief
and finds her way back to the ocean of life.

I am she who loves the magic of words
to inspire, empower, and heal.

I am she who is free to flower
in the garden of life.

TBI, They Said

Traumatic,
   shock wave to my
Brain,
   master computer
Injury,
   damage to my nerves.

A sentence
life-long
my nervous system
dismantled.
I piece it back
together,
  S
     L
       O
         W
           L
             Y.

Now, I say

   TBI

Transformed

     By

        Injury.

THANK YOU

for the challenge to recreate my life
after brain injury

for the gift of chaos
to generate new direction for my life

for the opportunity to find my anger
after the anarchy of a car wreck

for the chance to find
the denied part of myself
after my boundaries were shattered like glass

for the wake up call to attend my wounds,
to heal at a deeper level

for the experience of my children's love
when I came out of a coma
erasing any guilt for not being a perfect mother

for the injury to my left side, the happy side of my brain
so I could address the dark night in my soul
without interference from the light for a while

for a reason to go on living
creative urges to tell the story
to share and gain wisdom.

Thank you, God
for sending an angel with a message
that traumas are about transformation.

Resources for Transformation

Disclaimer:
The author has found the resources cited
in the following sections personally helpful,
but does not guarantee, approve,
or endorse the information or products
available on the included websites.

Journaling Prompts

RESEARCH DONE BY JAMES PENNEBAKER, PH.D., chair of the Department of Psychology at the University of Texas, demonstrates the positive effects that writing can have on healing. I personally found writing to be an enormous help in processing the emotional part of my own healing after traumatic brain injury.

I first learned of journaling sentence prompts to facilitate writing when I read Kay Adam's book *Journal to the Self.* Adams calls such writing prompts "Springboards" because like a swimming pool's diving board, "a Springboard launches you in a direction....its primary function is to get you into action!"

To use a journaling sentence prompt, start by writing the sentence prompt in your journal, or notebook, or anywhere you wish to write. Then continue writing whatever comes to your mind, without censoring it.

Following are the sample writing prompts that worked best for me in recovery.

I reclaim...

I am a woman/man who...

I am grateful for...

When I can't understand something, I feel...

What I want the world to know about brain injury is...

What do I care most about?

I am she/he who...

When I'm alone I feel...

I feel most sad about...

What makes me most angry is...

When I can't find words for what I want to say, I feel...

The biggest thing I lost is...and it makes me feel...

I'm proud of myself for...

Things that bring me comfort...

When I'm scared I want to...

I wish I could...

What I accomplished last week...

What brings me the most joy?

No one knows...

What I like about the new me is...

I dream...

TBI Resources

LISTED BELOW ARE THE RESOURCES that have been most helpful to me in my own recovery from traumatic brain injury.

TREATMENTS

Acupuncture:
> www.acufinder.com
> Resource for information on acupuncture, Chinese herbs and Asian medicine.

Adrenal Health:
> www.womentowomen.com & www.adrenalfatigue.org
> Information on subclinical adrenal dysfunction, also called adrenal imbalance or adrenal fatigue.

Amen Clinics:
> www.amenclinics.net
> Help for people with a wide range of issues who want a better brain and a better life.

Biocranial Institute:
> www.biocranialinstitute.com
> The Bio Craniopathic System of healthcare addresses disorders of the body's Master System, upon whose function depends that of all other bodily systems—circulatory, musculoskeletal, respiratory, endocrine, neurological, etc.

Brain State Conditioning:
> www.brainstatetech.com
> A holistic and noninvasive neurotechnology that guides a brain back to its natural, balanced state.

CranioSacral Therapy:
www.upledger.com
CranioSacral Therapy (also spelled "cranialsacral") is a
gentle, hands-on method of evaluating and enhancing
the functioning of a physiological body system called the
craniosacral system—comprised of the membranes and
cerebrospinal fluid that surround and protect the brain
and spinal cord—to improve the functioning of the central
nervous system.

EMDR Institute, Inc.:
www.emdr.com
EMDR (Eye Movement Desensitization and Reprocessing)
is a psychotherapy that enables people to heal from the
symptoms and emotional distress that are the result of
disturbing life experiences, including posttrraumatic stress
disorder.

Hyperbaric Oxygen Treatment:
HBOT chambers can usually be found at Autism Centers
for children in local communities.

Dr. Robert Kohn:
www.drrobertkohn.com
Dr. Kohn is a neuropsychiatrist who approaches each
patient as a whole, assessing symptoms using a biological-
psychological-social framework. Dr. Kohn refers people with
TBI to the University of Illinois, Chicago for Brain Spect
Scans.

Naturopathic Medicine:
www.naturopathic.org
The American Association of Naturopathic Physicians
(AANP) is the national professional society representing
licensed or licensable naturopathic physicians who are
graduates of four-year residential graduate programs.

Healthcare Practitioners

THE FOLLOWING IS A LIST of healthcare facilities and medical practitioners involved in my recovery.

Colorado:

Boulder Community Hospital,
Mapleton Rehabilitation Center: www.bch.org
Julie Stapleton, M.D., Neurotrauma Specialist:
http://www.juliestapletonmd.com

Illinois:

Brain Injury Clinic—Robert Kohn, D.O.:
www.braininjuryclinic.com & www.drrobertkohn.com
Dan Lippmann, L.C.S.W.—Emotional Transformation Therapy: www.wellness-innovations.com
Sylvia Lippmann, C.L.C.—Life Coach:
www.feelbetternow-ci.com
Marianjoy Outpatient Rehabilitation Services:
www.marianjoy.org
Alice Nixon, L.C.S.W.—specializes in PTSD and stress management, uses EMDR:
www.brainbreakthrough.com & www.letsaskalice.com
Rehabilitation Institute of Chicago:
www.ric.org
Kim Trager, D.C.—Applied Kinesiology, Cranialsacral Massage Therapy: www.tragerhealing.com
Sally VanCura, L.Ac, M.S.O.M.
Biocranial Therapy & acupuncture—www.herboria.com
Deborah Zelinsky, F.N.O.R.A, F.C.O.V.D.
www.mindeyeconnection.com
Optometrist whose practice emphasizes neuro-optometric rehabilitation by using the eye as a portal into brain function.

Minnesota:

Courage Center:
www.couragecenter.org
Hearthstone Institute—Darell M. Shaffer, M.D.:
www.hearthstoneinstitute.com
Thomas Bergquist, Ph.D.—Mayo Clinic Midwest Advocacy Project (Research Department):
www.mayoresearch.mayo.edu/mayo/research/staff/bergquist_tf.cfm
Paulette Hastings, B.A., Alina Janssen, B.A.—Brainwave Optimization:
www.neurostrength.com
Robert Karol, Ph.D., Karol Neuropsychological Service and Consulting:
11800 Singletree Ln #203
Eden Prairie, MN 55344
Minnesota Hyperbaric Treatment Center:
www.mnhyperbaric.org
John Nash, Ph.D.—psychologist, neurofeedback:
www.qeeg.com

Florida:

Jacqueline Riker, L.M.T.—Cranialsacral therapist:
http://rahnwyn.com

Support & Information Sites

Brain Injury Association of America:
www.biausa.org
The country's oldest and largest nationwide brain injury advocacy organization.
Brain Injury.com:
www.braininjury.com
Medical and legal information on brain injury.

Brain Injury Online:
www.brain-injury-online.com
A comprehensive source of information about living with an injured brain.

Brain Injury Resource Center:
www.headinjury.com/resources.htm
Traumatic Brain Injury resources and services.

Brainline.org:
www.brainline.org
BrainLine is a national multimedia project offering information and resources about preventing, treating, and living with TBI.

Centre for Neuro Skills®:
www.neuroskills.com
Information, services and products relating to traumatic brain injury, brain injury recovery and post-acute rehabilitation.

Dr. Diane®: www.health-helper.com
Dr. Diane is a licensed psychologist and neuropsychologist, board-certified in both health and sports psychology, who works with individuals and organizations worldwide to help them find solutions and resources. She is a survivor of a stroke and four TBIs, and the author of *Coping with Mild Traumatic Brain Injury* (Diane Roberts Stoler, Ed.D., 1997, Avery Trade Paperback).

Give Back: Road Maps to Recovery:
www.givebackorlando.com
GiveBack, Inc. is a recovery group for traumatic brain injury (TBI). Its purpose is not to help survivors to accept new lives that offer them limited options, but rather to help recoverers deal with their deficits, improve their functioning, become active, and regain self-control of their lives.

Health Journeys:
www.healthjourneys.com
Belleruth Naparstek, L.I.S.W. produces CDs with guided imagery for visualization that are very helpful in managing anxiety, depression, PTSD and other physical ailments.

International Society for Neurofeedback and Research (ISNR): www.isnr.org
The ISNR is a nonprofit member organization for professionals pursuing research and the promotion of self regulation of brain activity for healthier functioning.

Journal After Brain Injury:
www.barbarastahura.com
Barbara Stahura's website with link to her blog includes information about journaling for people with brain injury and their family caregivers.

Lash & Associates Publishing:
www.lapublishing.com
Leading source of information on brain injury in children, adolescents, adults and veterans.

National Institute of Neurological Disorders and Stroke (NINDS):
www.ninds.nih.gov
The mission of NINDS is to reduce the burden of neurological disease borne by every age group, every segment of society, and by people all over the world.

Realistic Hope:
www.realistichope.com
An online community intended for those touched by brain injury to learn, share, connect, collaborate and mentor others.

The Brain Injury Recovery Network:
> www.tbirecovery.org
> A nonprofit organization dedicated to helping survivors and families of brain and other serious injuries.

Traumatic Brain Injury Survival Guide:
> www.tbiguide.com
> The goal of this online book by Dr. Glen Johnson, clinical neuropsychologist, is to better prepare the head injured person and family for the long road ahead.

Resources for Writers

Kay Adams, L.P.C.—author, psychotherapist & founder of the **Center for Journal Therapy**:
www.journaltherapy.com & http://twinstitute.net

Linda Leedy Schneider, L.M.S.W., Writing Mentor—
http://www.pw.org/content/linda_leedy_schneider

About the Author

LOUISE MATHEWSON HOLDS A MASTER'S DEGREE in pastoral studies from Loyola University in Chicago. Her work has appeared in numerous publications, including *Wordgathering: Journal of Disability Poetry, Mochila Review, Boulder County Kid* and *Sasee* magazines, and the anthologies *Cup of Comfort—Vol. I* (Adams Media) and *Borderlines '08* (University of Portsmouth, United Kingdom). Most recently her work appears in *Mentor's Bouquet,* an anthology edited by Linda Leedy Schneider (Finishing Line Press, Fall 2009).

Louise has always loved to write about the sacred moments in everyday experiences, but today these experiences hold even deeper meaning. In February 2003 she emerged from a two-week coma following an auto accident in which she suffered a traumatic brain injury. Though she struggled at first, she resumed writing as soon as she was able. Today Louise lives with her husband in Eden Prairie, Minnesota, where she continues to write and recover.

About Pearlsong Press

PEARLSONG PRESS IS AN INDEPENDENT publishing company dedicated to providing books and resources that entertain while expanding perspectives on the self and the world. The company was founded by Peggy Elam, Ph.D., a psychologist and journalist, in 2003.

We encourage you to enjoy other Pearlsong Press books, which you can purchase at www.pearlsong.com or your favorite bookstore. Keep up with us through our blog at www.pearlsongpress.com.

FICTION:

The Falstaff Vampire Files—paranormal adventure by Lynne Murray
Larger Than Death—a Josephine Fuller mystery by Lynne Murray
Large Target—a Josephine Fuller mystery by Lynne Murray
The Season of Lost Children—a novel by Karen Blomain
Fallen Embers & *Blowing Embers*—Books 1 & 2 of The Embers
Series, paranormal romance by Lauri J Owen
The Fat Lady Sings—a young adult novel by Charlie Lovett
Syd Arthur—a novel by Ellen Frankel
Bride of the Living Dead—romantic comedy by Lynne Murray
Measure By Measure—a romantic romp with the fabulously fat by
Rebecca Fox & William Sherman
FatLand—a visionary novel by Frannie Zellman
The Program—a suspense novel by Charlie Lovett
The Singing of Swans—a novel about the Divine Feminine
by Mary Saracino

ROMANCE NOVELS & SHORT STORIES FEATURING BIG BEAUTIFUL HEROINES:

by Pat Ballard, the Queen of Rubenesque Romances:
Dangerous Love | *The Best Man* | *Abigail's Revenge*
Dangerous Curves Ahead: Short Stories | *Wanted: One Groom*
Nobody's Perfect | *His Brother's Child* | *A Worthy Heir*
by Rebecca Brock—*The Giving Season*
& by Judy Bagshaw—*At Long Last, Love: A Collection*

NONFICTION:

Talking Fat: Health vs. Persuasion in the War on Our Bodies—
nonfiction by Lonie McMichael, Ph.D.
ExtraOrdinary: An End of Life Story Without End—
memoir by Michele Tamaren & Michael Wittner
Love is the Thread: A Knitting Friendship by Leslie Moïse, Ph.D.
Fat Poets Speak: Voices of the Fat Poets' Society—Frannie Zellman, Ed.
Ten Steps to Loving Your Body (No Matter What Size You Are)
by Pat Ballard
Beyond Measure: A Memoir About Short Stature & Inner Growth
by Ellen Frankel
*Taking Up Space: How Eating Well & Exercising Regularly Changed
My Life* by Pattie Thomas, Ph.D. with Carl Wilkerson, M.B.A.
(foreword by Paul Campos, author of *The Obesity Myth*)
*Off Kilter: A Woman's Journey to Peace with Scoliosis, Her Mother & Her
Polish Heritage*—a memoir by Linda C. Wisniewski
Unconventional Means: The Dream Down Under
—a spiritual travelogue by Anne Richardson Williams
Splendid Seniors: Great Lives, Great Deeds—inspirational biographies
by Jack Adler

HEALING THE WORLD ONE BOOK AT A TIME

www.ingramcontent.com/pod-product-compliance
Lightning Source LLC
Chambersburg PA
CBHW022013090426
42741CB00007B/1017